FAT FROM FICTION

A CRITICAL LOOK AT DIETARY FATS AND WHY YOU SHOULD DITCH THE HEALTH GURUS AND LISTEN TO YOUR BODY

BY: JOEY LOTT

www.JoeyLottHealth.com

Publishing services provided by 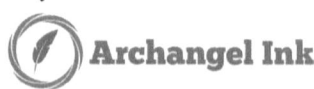 **Archangel Ink**

ISBN: 1518666566
ISBN-13: 978-1518666568

Table of Contents

Introduction

When it comes to dietary advice, there's often a lot of conflicting information. And in particular, there's been a lot of confusing information making headlines and best-selling books when it comes to dietary fat. What's the right thing to do? What should we be eating? What should we not be eating? Are the health gurus right? Which ones? In this book, we're going to take a closer look and see if we can find a sensible, sustainable, satisfying approach to dietary fat. Come along for the ride.

I came of age during the "fat-free" era of American dietary history. As a chubby kid, teased for the way my body looked, I fell prey to the fad. I took it to an extreme, eliminating as much dietary fat as I could from what I ate. At the time, of course, food companies were clambering for market share, and there was no shortage of fat-free varieties of popular foods, including Fat-Free Fig Newtons (which, if I recall correctly, actually weren't too bad) and nonfat frozen yogurt as a (less satisfying) stand-in for ice cream. Heck, those clever marketers even sold us "fat-free" fat. No, I'm not kidding. So big was the fad that some hotshot marketer got the idea that since the "serving size" was so small for cooking sprays, a technical loophole could allow them to promote the product as being "fat-free."

The "fat-free" phase of American history was extreme (not that most people took it to the extreme that I did), but for over half a century, we've had the less extreme (but thoroughly crazy-making) recommendations of the American Heart Association and the American Diabetic Association and even the U.S. Department of Agriculture (USDA). The purported public health advocacy organizations suggest simply that we all aim to reduce our overall dietary fat intake while giving *special* emphasis to reducing our intake of saturated fat. When we must eat dietary fat, these organizations advise that we eat polyunsaturated fat instead of saturated fat. In other words, butter is bad while soy oil is super, according to the advice doled out by these groups.

Somewhere along the line, some clever marketers hyped up the benefits of fish oils and we all started buying them in hopes that we could prevent heart attacks, strokes, cancer, and Alzheimer's, among other benefits attributed to the miracle oil. What was at one time largely an unprofitable by-product of the fishing industry grew to $425 million in sales in the U.S. in 2007. The growth has only intensified as sales in the U.S. jumped to a whopping $1.4 *billion* in 2012, according to Euromonitor International.

And yet along came the Weston A. Price Foundation's dietary recommendations ala *Nourishing Traditions* and the now-popular paleo diet movement, proclaiming loudly that saturated fat got a bad rap. (Ironically, Loren Cordain, arguably the originator of the modern paleo fad, never promoted saturated fat. Instead, he suggested that Paleolithic foods were likely naturally lower in saturated fat and total fat than modern foods. But be that as it may, the message about the guiltless nature of saturated fat has drowned out the original.) Although at first it seemed too good to be true ("You mean I can eat butter again?" people asked incredulously), the idea gained momentum and scientific support.

Now we're all mixed up. We've still got the diehards who claim that all dietary fat is bad—the Dr. McDougalls of the world. At the other extreme we have the "fat adapted" crowd of Mark Sisson and the ketogenic, nearly all-fat diet crowd who are livin' la vida low carb. We have doctors and nutritionists recommending that people should swap corn oil for butter to protect their hearts. And on the other hand we have those who shun not only all vegetable seed oils, but also chicken and pork because of their polyunsaturated fat content. Meanwhile, 10 percent of the population is guzzling fish oil like it's going out of style. Yet some niche dietary pundits warn that fish oil is deadly poison.

Who's right? Who's wrong? Is there any way to make sense of all of this? What should we eat? What should we avoid?

Relax. I'm going to sort fat, er, *fact* from fiction, and we'll see if we can make sense of this whole mess. It's both a whole lot more complicated and a whole lot less complicated than it seems.

In what follows, we'll look one by one at topics such as vegetable seed oils, fish oil, saturated fat, low fat, and high fat. We'll see what research has *really* revealed about these topics, so you can make educated and healthful decisions.

Understanding Fat Basics

Before we discuss the ins and outs of different types of fats and various dietary approaches to fat intake, let's first look at the basics of dietary fats and terminology that we'll use throughout the book. You have probably heard many of these terms, but you may not know exactly what they mean or why they are significant.

We all hopefully know what dietary fat is in general. Whether we're talking about butter, coconut oil, cocoa butter, sunflower seed oil, soy oil, or fish oil, they all have a similar quality to them. We recognize them because we can eat them or use them for other uses such as skin care (though take a tip from the pros and don't use fish oil as a hand moisturizer—cocoa butter's your better bet) and because they have an oily or greasy feel to them.

Fats also play important roles in the health inside of our bodies. Consider for a second that the human brain is composed primarily of fat and the entire nervous system is insulated by fat. And fats serve as an important energy source as well. Fat is essential to life. Without it, you'd die.

Dietary fats can obviously serve as a source of fats for the body, but fats are so important for health that the body has a backup system. Through a process called de novo lipogenesis (which is Latin for "new fat creation," but if you say "de novo lipogenesis," you'll sound more in the know), our bodies can create new fats that it needs—at least for *most* types of fats. There are a few types of fats that our bodies cannot make. Those types of fats are therefore called "essential" fats because we must obtain them from food. As we'll see, there is some disagreement about how much of these fats are truly needed. But small amounts of these types of fats appear in just about every type of natural food, and in free living humans, no evidence of deficiencies have been demonstrated.

So what we've seen is that fats are a category of nutrients that share some similar qualities. But they are not all the same. You can think of it this way: All automobiles are similar, but there are significant differences between the different types of automobiles. For example, a Honda Civic and an 18-wheeler both have engines and wheels, but the sizes of the engines and the number of wheels differ significantly. And each performs tasks slightly differently. The 18-wheeler is great for hauling big loads on the highway, but it doesn't perform so great in your driveway. The Honda, on the other hand, is great in town, but stick a suitcase in the back and it can't make it up the hill. Hopefully that metaphor helps to explain how, similarly, different types of fats, while sharing many things in common, are at the same time quite different.

What is it that makes all fats *similar*? Their similarity is that they are composed of building blocks called fatty acids. Those fatty acids all have a similar structure. They are all composed of chains of carbon atoms with hydrogens attached to the carbons. Don't worry. I'm not going to get all "sciencey" on you just yet. All that means is that the building blocks of fatty acids are the same regardless of the types of fatty acids.

All that differs is the length of the chain (i.e., the number of carbon atoms) and the types of bonds (either single or double) between the carbon atoms. Those differences account for whether a fatty acid is the Civic or the 18-wheeler of the fat world.

In a broad sense, fats are classified as being of three types: saturated, monounsaturated, or polyunsaturated. These classifications are based only on the types of bonds in the fatty acids. Fatty acids that have no double bonds are saturated. Those that have a single (mono) double bond are monounsaturated. And those with multiple (poly) double bonds are polyunsaturated. Double bonds make fats less stable.

With 100 percent single bonds, saturated fats are the most stable, and they are generally solid at room temperature. For example, butter, which contains a lot of saturated fat, is solid at room temperature, as is coconut oil (which is more highly saturated than butter). And because of their stability, we can typically store highly saturated fats at room temperature without fear of them going bad. That's why there is no need to refrigerate coconut oil.

Monounsaturated fats are the middle ground. They are less stable than saturated fats but more stable than polyunsaturated fats. That's because monounsaturated fats, as the name suggests, have exactly *one* double bond with the rest being single. They are generally liquid at room temperature, but at cool temperatures (such as in the refrigerator) they will become slightly more viscous. Olive oil is the classic example of a fat that is mostly monounsaturated. Most highly monounsaturated fats can be stored at room temperature but not for as long as highly saturated fats. For example, you can safely store coconut oil for a few years at room temperature (assuming you don't get water or bits of food in it or expose it to strong light, which will cause it to go bad). However, olive oil, which is mostly monounsaturated, will only stay good for a few months at room temperature. (Incidentally, other than those who believe that all dietary fat is bad, very few people hold anything against monounsaturated fat. So we won't be talking about it in too much detail in this book.)

Polyunsaturated fats are the least stable of the fats. They go rancid easily. They are liquid at room temperature and when refrigerated. Storage of highly polyunsaturated fats varies from type to type. If the oil is unrefined, most will be best stored in the refrigerator. For example, most fish oils and flaxseed oils are best in the refrigerator to reduce the rate at which the oils go rancid. However, as we'll see, most highly polyunsaturated fats (seed oils) are typically highly processed and refined. That can extend the shelf life before they clearly go rancid (though many argue that almost all industrially produced seed oils are oxidized [made rancid] in the production process).

When it comes to polyunsaturated fats, there are two main sub-categories. One is omega 6 polyunsaturated fats found in large amounts in nuts, seeds, and their oils. Many modern "vegetable" oils (which are really seed oils) such as soy and corn oils are very high in omega 6 fatty acids.

The other sub-category is omega 3 fats. There are some select seeds that are high in some types of omega 3 fats. For example, flaxseed is high in an omega 3 fat called alpha-linolenic acid. However, fish are the most common source of omega 3 fats, which is one of the reasons why fish oils are hyped as nutritional supplements.

There's much more to fats than this brief overview may suggest, but this is the foundation. As we continue, we'll look more in depth at the different types of fats and what the health implications of them might be.

Be aware that in natural foods none of these types of fat ever exist in isolation. There are no *purely* saturated, monounsaturated, or polyunsaturated fats found in real foods. For example, coconut oil is one of the most highly saturated fats found in common foods. And yet it also contains about 6 percent monounsaturated fat and 3 percent polyunsaturated fat. On the other extreme, flax oil, which can be up to 90 percent polyunsaturated, also contains a complement of saturated and monounsaturated fats.

Vegetable Seed Oils

There are a few traditional vegetable seed oils such as sesame. However, the vast majority of vegetable seed oils have only been extracted for food for a short time in history. They include soy, corn, safflower, sunflower, flaxseed, peanut, cottonseed, and canola as well as a few other less popular varieties.

Obviously, all vegetable seed oils (from now on, simply seed oils) are not equal. There are variations among them. For example, safflower oil is approximately 75 percent polyunsaturated while peanut is only 32 percent polyunsaturated. And while almost all of the polyunsaturated fat in corn or cottonseed oil is linoleic acid, an omega 6 fatty acid, around 80 percent of the polyunsaturated fat in flaxseed oil is alpha-linolenic acid, an omega 3 fatty acid.

However, what the majority of seed oils have in common is that they are high in polyunsaturated fats with a significant amount of that being an omega 6 fatty acid. The other thing they have in common is that most of them are extracted in part or in full using a solvent such as hexane and then refined. In other words, they are highly processed, often using non-food substances that are later removed. (Obviously, expeller-pressed seed oils, such as some flaxseed oil, are *not* solvent extracted, though they may or may not be refined. But the majority of seed oils for sale are solvent extracted and refined.)

The history of seed oils is an interesting one. Until the 20th century, seed oils were virtually unheard of for food. There are a few notable exceptions. For example, sesame oil, which is *relatively* easily expressed from the seeds (but not anywhere *near* as easy as it is to obtain more traditional fats like coconut oil, lard, or butter) has been used in very small amounts in food for thousands of years. But otherwise, most seed oils were simply not accessible in any volume because their extraction requires modern industrial technology and chemical inputs.

Flaxseed oil (also known as linseed oil), like sesame oil, is *relatively* easily expressed naturally, and it was used for paint for over a thousand years. For example, there is evidence of seed oil paints (likely flaxseed) being used in the 6th century, and specific written mention of flaxseed oil for paint appears in the 12th century. But as far as we know, by and large, people weren't eating it. That didn't happen until the latter part of the 20th century when flaxseed paints were largely replaced by chemical paints and the flaxseed industry sought a new market.

The first major introduction of seed oils into the human diet began in the late 19th century, though the fact was hidden from people because it was known that no one wanted to eat seed oils. In the middle of the 19th century, a man named William Fee invented a machine to press oil from cottonseeds. Prior to that, cottonseed had been a troublesome by-product of the huge cotton industry. But Fee's invention allowed for the seeds to be pressed into oil. At the same time, European population growth and economic conditions led to a shortage of whale oil and lard used to light lamps. The cotton industry took advantage and sold cottonseed oil to the Europeans, creating a market for the product.

But when the market dried up due to the introduction of cheaper petroleum oils, the cottonseed producers needed to find a new market. In the late 19th century, it was discovered that cottonseed oil was being used as an adulterant to lard. The volume of lard being sold eclipsed the amount of lard that could be produced from the total number of pigs. When this was found out, cottonseed oil prices plummeted.

Proctor and Gamble saw an opportunity. With cottonseed oil prices low, the company grabbed up the product and used industrial processes to artificially hydrogenate it (we'll discuss this process shortly). The result was a product called Crisco. Crisco was marketed as an alternative to lard, which was the dominant cooking fat at the time. Proctor and Gamble advertised Crisco as being "a healthier alternative" based not on any sort of science but purely to make the otherwise unappealing product attractive. And attractive it became—though likely more because of the low price than the supposed health benefits. Cottonseed oil began to replace other traditional fats largely due to Crisco.

A few decades later, soybeans began to rise to fame, and due to major industrial interest in soy and the relative dwindling of the cotton industry in the U.S., soy oil prices began to drop below those of cottonseed oil. As a result, soy oil came to be the new favorite seed oil, and major manufacturers of seed oil products such as Proctor and Gamble replaced cottonseed oil with soy oil in their products.

In the 1950s, Ancel Keys, the man famous for inventing K-rations and conducting the landmark Minnesota Starvation Experiment, found what he believed was a strong correlation between saturated fat intake and heart disease. He eventually gained influence with the American Heart Association (AHA) and, beginning in 1961, the AHA began to recommend (based, apparently, primarily on Keys' recommendations) that Americans should reduce their consumption of saturated fats from traditional foods such as butter and lard. This was a major shot in the arm for the seed oil industry because now claims of "heart healthy" soy or corn oil could be made without challenge.

The next big milestone in seed oil production and sales was the development of canola oil in the 1970s. Canola is produced from a specially bred variety of rapeseed, which is a brassica seed. Rapeseed had never been useful as an edible oil because it naturally contains toxins and has an unpleasant taste. However, the new variety had been bred to have low toxins, and it could be fully refined, bleached, and deodorized to remove any unpalatable qualities. Canola oil had the advantage of having a higher monounsaturated fat content than soy oil and also having an improved, less viscous texture. Prior to the invention of canola, no one ate rapeseed oil in any quantities. But after the U.S. Food and Drug Administration (FDA) approved the oil for food use in 1985, sales began to rise rapidly.

Beginning around the turn of the century (1900), Americans were eating practically no seed oils. With the aggressive marketing of cottonseed oil products, however, Americans were eating about five kilograms of seed oils each per year by 1919. By 1959, the amount had doubled. And by 1999, Americans were eating nearly *six times* as much seed oil as they had in 1919.[1]

The implications of the changes in seed oil consumption are still being debated, and we'll look at that in more detail in just a moment, but what is quite certain is that the huge increase in seed oil consumption and the reduction in traditional fats such as lard and tallow has dramatically altered the fatty acid composition of diets in North America and in many places worldwide.

Consider for a moment the fat composition of traditional fats like lard, tallow, or butter. The following shows the average composition (in terms of saturated, monounsaturated, and polyunsaturated fats) of these three. (Composition will vary depending on breed, diet, and lifestyle of the animals, so these are just some rough figures.)

- **Lard**—41 percent saturated, 47 percent monounsaturated, 12 percent polyunsaturated
- **Tallow**—48 percent saturated, 50 percent monounsaturated, 2 percent polyunsaturated

---

[1] Cordain et al. Origins and evolution of the Western diet: health implications for the 21st Century. American Journal of Clinical Nutrition. 2005; 81(2): 341-354.

- **Butterfat**—66 percent saturated, 30 percent monounsaturated, 4 percent polyunsaturated

Now compare those numbers to the composition of some popular seed oils:

- **Soy oil**—15 percent saturated, 24 percent monounsaturated, 61 percent polyunsaturated
- **Safflower oil**—9 percent saturated, 13 percent monounsaturated, 78 percent polyunsaturated
- **Corn oil**—13 percent saturated, 25 percent monounsaturated, 62 percent polyunsaturated
- **Cottonseed oil**—27 percent saturated, 19 percent monounsaturated, 54 percent polyunsaturated

As you can hopefully see, until the 1900s, Americans (and most people worldwide) were relying primarily on traditional dietary fats in their foods. As a result, in general, the fatty acid composition of foods was skewed *heavily* toward saturated and monounsaturated fats with very small amounts of polyunsaturated fats. Even in cultures in which the people have traditionally eaten a lot of oily fish (which is relatively high in polyunsaturated fat), the majority of the fatty acids were from saturated or monounsaturated types. For example, the fatty acid composition of salmon oil is as follows:

- **Salmon oil**—20 percent saturated, 55 percent monounsaturated, 25 percent polyunsaturated

Also, as we'll see shortly, many traditional foods—even those high in polyunsaturated fat—tend to have low omega 6 to omega 3 ratios.

The trend toward increased consumption of seed oils has dramatically reversed the proportions of saturated to polyunsaturated fats. Seed oils are typically very high in polyunsaturated fats while being low in saturated and monounsaturated fats. And the omega 6 to omega 3 ratio of most seed oils is extremely high.

How much has this shift affected the diets of Americans and others worldwide? Well, in 2003, over 80 percent of all edible oil consumption in the U.S. was from soy oil. Canola oil came in at a distant second. Then cottonseed oil.[2]

In 1900, American soy oil consumption per capita was a big fat zilch. In 1909, that number increased to 0.02 pounds per person. In 1999, the per capita consumption of soy oil in the U.S. was 25 pounds.

In the following figure, you can see a graphical representation that clearly demonstrates the shift since 1900. Using data from the USDA, I have charted reported consumption of butter and soy oil in the U.S. per person. As you can see, the latter has essentially replaced the former and then some.

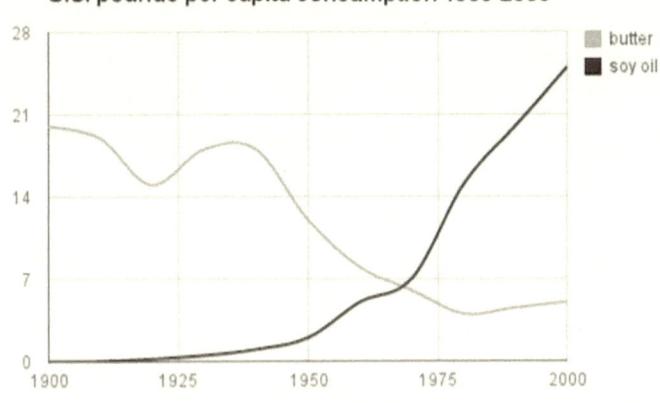

U.S. pounds per capita consumption 1900-2000

But what are the implications of this change? That is a matter we'll look at shortly.

---

[2] U.S. Census Bureau. Data available at
http://www.soystats.com/2004/page_23.htm.

Hydrogenation

One of the rather certain harmful effects of the increase in seed oil consumption is due to the *manner* in which many of the seed oils are processed. Of all the research into the health effects of seed oils, the negative consequences of partial hydrogenation are the clearest. In fact, the consensus in this regard is so strong that many states and even entire countries have effectively banned the use of partially hydrogenated oils.

The process of hydrogenation alters the physical structure of fats, raising the melting point. The result is that liquid seed oils can be made solid at room temperature by adding hydrogen atoms, a process called hydrogenation. Seed oil producers like this because it increases the desirability of their products. It improves the texture, the consistency, and stability of the product. Liquid soy or canola oil can be converted into margarine and sold as butter substitutes.

Hydrogenation of polyunsaturated oils was first patented in 1902 by a German chemist named Wilhelm Normann. In 1909, Proctor and Gamble purchased the rights to use the patent with plans to take advantage of depressed cottonseed oil prices. And, as stated earlier, in 1911, Proctor and Gamble began to produce and aggressively market Crisco, which was (and is) a hydrogenated oil product intended to replace lard and butter for Americans.

A precedent for butter replacement had been established nearly half a century previous in France. Napoleon III had issued a challenge for the creation of a butter substitute to feed the "working class and the Navy." A French chemist by the name of Mège-Mouriès succeeded by mixing beef tallow with buttermilk, a product he called oleomargarine. Thus, margarine was born. However, prior to the discovery of the hydrogenation of oils, margarine had been produced using naturally occurring, traditional fats such as tallow. With hydrogenation, seed oil margarine could be produced for dirt cheap in comparison.

The process of hydrogenation, as the name implies, adds hydrogen to a substance—in this case, oils. When hydrogen is added to polyunsaturated fats, the result is that the bond structure between carbon atoms in the fatty acid changes. Unsaturated fats have double bonds between some of the carbon atoms in fatty acids. The double bonds have at least two effects. For one, they decrease the stability of the fatty acids, making them more susceptible to rancidity. For another, they lower the melting point so that unsaturated fats are liquid at room temperature. Since polyunsaturated fats have more double bonds than monounsaturated fats and saturated fats (which have no double bonds), polyunsaturated fats are the least stable and have the lowest melting point of the three types of fats.

Poor stability (easily going rancid) and low melting point are not good selling points when it comes to edible fats. People want fats that will keep well and that can be spread, mixed, and used for baking with ease (like butter or coconut oil, for example) Liquid seed oils don't meet those criteria. But hydrogenation reduces the double bonds and converts unsaturated fats into *saturated* fats.

In fact, if hydrogenation is done fully, the resultant fat is fully saturated. However, in practice, no food products are fully hydrogenated because the resultant product would have an unappealing texture and the melting point would be too high. A better texture and workability is achieved when only *some* of the double bounds are altered. So food chemists at companies like

Proctor and Gamble found that it was necessary to control the hydrogenation process so that it would only be *partial*. Some of the polyunsaturated fats are converted to saturated, but many are not. Those with the fewest double bonds become saturated, but those with the most double bonds remain unsaturated.

The trouble with partial hydrogenation of seed oils is that it results in a large number of altered unsaturated fats that have configurations that are not found in natural foods. And it is increasingly clear that these unnatural fats are harmful to health.

You may have heard of the phrase "trans fats" as it has gained popularity in the past decade or so. But most of us don't know what it means. In order to understand this, I'll have to briefly go into more detail about the chemical structure of fats. Bear with me. I'll keep it simple.

Fatty acids are composed of chains of carbon and hydrogen. The following image shows one way to represent the chemical structure of fatty acids. The top image shows a snippet of an unsaturated fatty acid. The lines represent chemical bonds. You can see that most of them are single bonds (indicated by a single line). But between two of the carbon atoms (represented by the letter C) there's a double bond (indicated by double lines looking like an equals sign). Where there are double bonds, the carbon atoms on either side of the bond will only be bonded to one hydrogen atom (H), which is different than single bonded carbons that bond to two hydrogen atoms. That sounds complicated, but hopefully the image is clear.

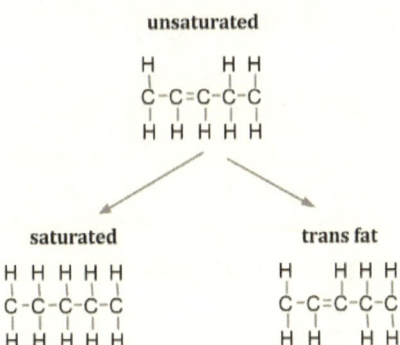

The lines with arrows represent the process of hydrogenation. Remember, this is only supposed to be a snippet of a fatty acid carbon chain. So theoretically, there could be only the one double bond, but there may also be other double bonds elsewhere in the fatty acid. If there is only one double bond and just two hydrogen atoms are added, the result is a full hydrogenation or a full saturation of the fatty acid as shown in the lower left representation. But if there are multiple double bonds and not enough hydrogen atoms are added to fully saturate the fatty acid, the bonds that don't receive hydrogen atoms will twist. The result is that at the double bond, the hydrogens on either side will be on flip sides of one another (trans, meaning across) instead of the normal position, being on the same side (cis, meaning same side).

This may seem like a trivial alteration. However, it turns out that it has huge implications. Trans fats that are produced through partial hydrogenation are similar enough to normal fats that human bodies will make use of them. However, once these trans fats are used in the body, they fail to work as the body expects. The result is metabolic derangement.

Incidentally, there are very few naturally occurring trans fats. Two that are known are conjugated linoleic acid (CLA) and vaccenic acid, both of which appear in the meat and dairy from ruminants and which may be produced naturally by so-called beneficial bacteria in your digestive system. However, both CLA and vaccenic acid have been shown to be either likely harmless or possibly beneficial. Research into the effects on human health of naturally occurring trans fats is still a relatively new field. Presumably, however, humans have co-evolved with these naturally occurring fats and have few if any problems with them.

However, unlike naturally occurring trans fats, the trans fats produced during partial hydrogenation have been found to be consistently linked to cardiovascular disease risk. They have also been linked to type 2 diabetes, liver problems, abdominal fat, and depression.

The strongest association, as indicated, is with cardiovascular disease. A number of studies have shown this connection, and a 2006 review from Harvard [3] found that there is a strong association between trans fat consumption and heart disease. Perhaps one of the strongest indictments of trans fats comes from a major, long-term study that has shown that for every 2 percent increase in trans fats in humans there is a *doubling* of risk for heart disease

All in all, it has become increasingly clear that trans fats produced by partial hydrogenation are likely bad for human health. As a result, governments have been slowly enacting laws that limit the sale of food products containing significant amounts of trans fats. Naturally occurring trans fats make up a very small percentage of the foods in which they appear. However, the trans fat content of partially hydrogenated oils is often very high. For example, partially hydrogenated soy oil is about 40 percent trans fats.

In 2003, Denmark was the first country to pass laws to restrict trans fats. The law allows for no more than 2 percent of any food ingredient to be composed of trans fats. The Danish law has the

---

[3] Mozaffarian et al. Trans fatty acids and cardiovascular disease. New England Journal of Medicine. 2006; 354(15): 1601-1613.

practical effect of removing partially hydrogenated oils from the food supply.

Subsequent to the Danish legislation, other European governments followed suit. Switzerland, Austria, Iceland, and Sweden have all either passed similar laws or have similar laws pending.

In the United States, the FDA created a regulation requiring that all food products list trans fat content on the label. And in 2013, the FDA determined that trans fats are *not* generally recognized as safe. That *could* result in changes at the federal level that would effectively ban partially hydrogenated oils from foods, but as of this writing that hasn't happened yet.

What *has* happened in the U.S. is that municipalities and states have passed laws regarding trans fats. A number of U.S. cities, including Boston, New York, Chicago, and Philadelphia, have passed legislation limiting or banning trans fats from partially hydrogenated oils in restaurants or in stores. A handful of counties have also passed similar laws. And the state of California has banned the use of partially hydrogenated trans fats in restaurants since 2010.

As a result of the increasingly negative views of trans fats, food manufacturers and vendors are beginning to phase out partially hydrogenated oils. That's very good news. But the century-long experiment with large amounts of trans fats in the food we ate may leave a legacy. The removal of those trans fats will hopefully shed some light on some matters that have puzzled many people for decades. The rise of trans fats closely parallels the rise in cardiovascular disease, increased fatness, and other conditions that are associated with metabolic derangement. Will the removal of those trans fats reverse the trends? That is yet to be seen. To date, the *only* strong evidence linking trans fats to specific health problems is regarding heart disease. Other proposed connections may not even actually exist, so I wouldn't hold my breath expecting trans fats elimination to be the magic cure for all ills. At the same time, I'd certainly suggest that minimizing unnatural trans fats in your diet is probably a good idea.

Omega 6

You'll recall that polyunsaturated fats fall into two sub-categories: omega 6 and omega 3. Let's first take a look at omega 6 fats.

There are eleven known omega 6 fatty acids. Most of them are fairly obscure and poorly researched. And as far as we know, *most* of them are rarely found in the foods that we eat. There are just a handful that show up in significant amounts, and those will be the ones we'll look at in more detail.

The most abundant omega 6 fatty acid in food is called linoleic acid. Conventionally, linoleic acid is considered to be an essential fatty acid because small amounts are needed by the human body, but we are not capable of synthesizing it as we are many other fatty acids. And humans are capable of converting linoleic acid to other omega 6 fats, so technically, it's the only essential omega 6 fatty acid.

How much linoleic acid is necessary for health maintenance? Well, according to the United States National Academy of Sciences (the organization that defines recommended daily allowances), adult women need *at least* 12 grams and adult men need *at least* 17 grams of linoleic acid per day. Based on the (low) calorie recommendations of 2000 and 2500 calories, respectively, that means the recommended intake of linoleic acid is about 6 percent of total calories. The U.S. is not alone in these recommendations. Other countries have very similar recommendations, with some being even higher.

As we've seen, the dominant sources of dietary fats prior to the 1900s were foods such as coconut oil, lard, butter, and tallow. Modern lard, butter, and tallow are typically higher in linoleic acid than they would have been for most of human history because exclusive grain feeding increases the linoleic acid levels. But using modern values we get about 3 percent for both butter and tallow and anywhere from 6 to 10 percent for lard (depending on breed and other factors). And coconut oil has only about 2 percent linoleic acid.

At those levels, it would be necessary to eat 170 grams or more of lard or 567 grams of butter or tallow or 850 grams of coconut oil per day to eat 17 grams of linoleic acid. Even allowing that other foods eaten in normal amounts likely available to people for much of human history (nuts, seeds, poultry, grain, etc.) could provide a few grams of linoleic acid per day and reduce the amount that would need to be obtained from lard, butter, tallow, or other similar fats, it's kind of hard to believe that our ancestors were eating that much fat. I mean, 567 grams of butter is about 5 sticks of butter *per day*, which is pushing 4000 calories in butter alone.

So even on the surface, something doesn't add up with those recommendations. If we really needed that much linoleic acid every day, then humans wouldn't have survived all these generations with such huge deficiencies.

Modern seed oils are a novelty when it comes to linoleic acid in the human diet. Soy oil contains about 51 percent linoleic acid, so it is only necessary to eat 33 grams of soy oil to consume 17 grams of linoleic acid. And safflower oil can contain up to 79 percent linoleic acid, so it is only necessary to eat 22 grams of safflower oil to consume 17 grams of linoleic acid. Modern seed oils make it quite easy to obtain large amounts of linoleic acid, but before the1900s, it seems unlikely that the majority of people (who were obviously successful enough in health in order to reproduce effectively) were eating anything even approaching the recommended amount of linoleic acid.

Based simply on these observations, it might be tempting to disregard the recommended intake for linoleic acid as excessive. But before we do that, let's look at how the recommendation came to be. Was it due to rigorous study looking at how much linoleic acid is truly necessary for human health? Nope. It was not. Instead, it was based on self-reported survey data. Statisticians determined that 12 grams of linoleic acid is the average amount of self-reported linoleic acid healthy women ate while healthy men ate 17 grams. But only until age 50. After that, healthy women ate 11 grams and healthy men ate 14 grams (which are the official recommendations for people over 50).

Still, as we'll see in a minute, there is a fairly large body of evidence that suggests that increasing linoleic acid in the diet improves human health. Let's look at that next.

Linoleic Acid Improves Heart Health?

In 1929, George and Mildred Burr performed a study[4] in which they found that feeding rats a diet that consisted only of highly purified casein (protein) and sugar along with purified vitamins produced hair loss, scaly skin, and damage to the tail. (I'm guessing it also devastated those poor rats' appetites. I mean, that sounds like a rather unpleasant diet.) They reasoned that it must be due to a deficiency of some fat.

The next year, the Burrs published another paper detailing their further investigation into the matter.[5] The Burrs reported on what they viewed as the "cure" for the fat-free condition they were able to produce in the rats. Not surprisingly, giving the rats dietary fat was the cure. However, the Burrs noted that fats highest in linoleic acid produced the fastest cure. It is of note, however, that one of the indicators of the cure working (apart from improvement in skin and hair) was *rapid weight gain*. In other words, the greater the linoleic acid in the diet, the greater the weight gain.

Subsequent studies, such as those conducted by a man named Holman who had been an associate of the Burrs, went further to

---

[4] Burr GO and Burr MM. A new deficiency disease produced by rigid exclusion of fat from the diet. Journal of Biological Chemistry. 1929; 82: 345-367.

[5] Burr GO and Burr MM. On the nature and role of the fatty acids essential in nutrition. Journal of Biological Chemistry. 1930. 86; 587-621.

demonstrate that linoleic acid is essential for rats. Using purified fatty acids, Holman was able to demonstrate that only linoleic acid produced the cure for the fat-free condition.[6]

In 1998, Holman published a paper[7] in which he describes the evolution of the idea that linoleic acid is essential for humans. In that paper, he begins by citing the Burr and Burr experiments with rats. But the first study on the matter in humans was in 1938 with a study that attempted to reproduce the effects by feeding a single man a low-fat diet for six months. The outcome was no detectable negative alterations as the result of the low-fat diet.

Clearly, however, the 1938 study was flawed. It had only one participant and failed to restrict the diet to no fat. The next study Holman references is a 1970 case study of an infant who was placed on intravenous feeding shortly after birth because part of her intestines had been surgically removed. She was fed a fat-free preparation, and it was observed that she developed skin lesions after three months. Her skin was analyzed and found to be low in polyunsaturated fatty acids. This was taken as evidence that she developed skin lesions due to a deficiency in polyunsaturated fatty acids. Unfortunately, the girl died. We will never know whether she was suffering from a polyunsaturated fat deficiency or perhaps she was simply very sick, no doubt, in part due to having had part of her intestines removed.

Holman next references a case study from the same time period. This case study is of a 78-year-old woman who was also placed on fat-free intravenous feeding following having part of her intestines surgically removed. After the first month, she began to develop dermatitis that was not relieved by applying corn oil to the skin. Tests showed her to be low in

---

[6] Ray Peat has argued that the deficiency was not linoleic acid, but rather vitamin B6, which hadn't yet been discovered. I'm not sure he's right, but it's certainly an interesting consideration.

[7] Holman RT. The slow discovery of the importance of omega 3 fatty acids in human health. *Journal of Nutrition*. 1998; 128(2); 4275-4335.

polyunsaturated fatty acids when compared to other people. After seven months, she died of an infection.

That is the total of the evidence Holman, one of the leading proponents of the essential nature of linoleic acid, presents regarding the matter. It's not terribly convincing. But at the same time, there certainly does seem to be some evidence that a diet in which linoleic acid is completely absent may be problematic. At the very least, I'd suggest that if you happen to meet someone who is on total parenteral nutrition after having part of his or her intestines removed, recommend that a completely fat-free plan may not be ideal.

However, for everyone else it may be a moot point so long as a person is eating *real food* instead of receiving intravenous feeding. Why? Because most foods contain *some* linoleic acid, even if only in trace amounts. Remember that the Burrs were able to create the deficiency symptoms when placing rats on a highly purified diet in which all traces of fat were removed. (In fact, the process the Burrs went through to ensure that absolutely no traces of fat were to be found in the rats' food is a bit obsessive.) But in real foods, no such refinement is ever seen. For example, white rice, which has had most of the fat content removed along with the bran still contains about 150 mg of linoleic acid per serving. Brown rice has about three times as much. And just about *any* kind of natural fat, including butter, tallow, olive oil, and so forth, have modest amounts of linoleic acid. Furthermore, we simply don't see an epidemic of diseases among populations that stick to traditional diets that would be "deficient" in linoleic acid according to current recommendations.

My argument, therefore, is not that linoleic acid is not needed for health, but rather that the amounts needed are provided by any diet that provides adequate calories from a variety of natural foods and food groups.

Still, the National Academy of Science recommends that adults eat 12 or 17 grams of linoleic acid every day to avoid deficiency. The AHA recommends up to 10 percent of calories come from linoleic acid (which is nearly double the National

Academy of Science recommendations, which would be a *lot* of coconut oil) but for a different reason than the National Academy of Science. The AHA has done its homework and in 2009 published a paper [8] reviewing the relevant studies that demonstrated that increasing linoleic acid intake is associated with lower risk of cardiovascular disease events (heart attacks, strokes, etc.). (Interestingly, however, and not that this necessarily colors the findings, the AHA paper's lead author received "significant" financial support from corporations with a vested interest in selling linoleic acid.)

The AHA cites 60 controlled human studies that showed that increasing linoleic acid intake improved *markers* of cardiovascular health. And while those studies are very well designed and provide some potentially useful information, the authors admit that *markers* (i.e., test results and numbers) aren't always good predictors of actual outcomes. In other words, it is possible that studies could show that feeding people more linoleic acid will reduce their cholesterol levels, but ultimately that doesn't prove that feeding linoleic acid will result in fewer heart attacks.

The rest of the studies that are cited in the paper provide a confusing picture. Many of the studies had glaring errors. And the results of many of the cohort studies showed no association between linoleic acid and cardiovascular disease whatsoever. Overall, the authors conclude that the studies suggest a "modest benefit" of linoleic acid intake on cardiovascular disease.

The AHA's analysis is not without evidence to the contrary, though. In a recent analysis of an Australian study,[9] the authors found that men who increased their linoleic acid intake to 15 percent of calories in the study actually died more frequently than

---

[8] Harris et al. Omega-6 fatty acids and risk for cardiovascular disease. *Circulation.* 2009; 119: 902-907.

[9] Ramsden et al. Use of dietary linoleic acid for secondary prevention of coronary heart disease and death: evaluation of recovered data from the Sydney Diet Heart Study and updated meta-analysis. *British Medical Journal.* 2013; 346: e8707

the men who were on a much lower linoleic acid diet. They died more frequently from all causes as well as from heart disease. However, the increase in linoleic acid in the diets of the men in the study may have included trans fats, which may have complicated the results.

Another piece of evidence that is contrary to the findings of the AHA is the fact that Israel is the country with the highest per capita consumption of linoleic acid in the world and yet also has one of the highest rates of cardiovascular disease.[10] That doesn't prove that linoleic acid is the cause of cardiovascular disease, of course. But it does call into question the supposedly protective effects of linoleic acid when the country with the highest consumption also has high rates of the very conditions that it is supposed to protect against.

And what's more, one of the lead researchers whose studies were used by the AHA to claim that higher omega 6 intake is healthy, Christopher Ramsden of the National Institutes of Health, has since argued that the AHA has misrepresented his findings and that recommendations for higher omega 6 intake might actually *increase* cardiovascular disease risk.[11]

So hopefully you can see that the linoleic acid story is a complicated one. Should you be eating more or less of it? Stay with me, and we'll sort through this some more. Most of what we hear about these matters are simple sound bites. "Lower saturated fat." "Eat more vegetable oil." But those sound bites are overly simple. In order to make good decisions about these things, we need to rely on something more than sound bites.

---

[10] Yam et al. Diet and disease - the Israeli paradox: possible dangers of a high omega-6 polyunsaturated fatty acid diet. *Israel Journal of Medical Sciences.* 1996; 32(11): 1134-1143.

Berry EM. Are diets high in omega-6 polyunsaturated fatty acids unhealthy? *European Heart Journal Supplements.* 2001; 3(Supplement D): D37-D41.

[11] Ramsden et al. n-6 fatty acid-specific and mixed polyunsaturated dietary interventions have different effects on CHD risk: a meta-analysis of randomized controlled trials. *British Journal of Medicine.* 2010; 104(11): 1586-1600.

Arachidonic Acid

In recent years, some people have speculated that increasing linoleic acid may be harmful because it may increase inflammation. This theory is speculative and based on the fact that one of the ways that the body can use linoleic acid is to convert it to arachidonic acid, which is the other main omega 6 fatty acid of interest.

Arachidonic acid is the building block of many important substances in the body. Some of those substances are inflammatory, which has given arachidonic acid a bad name. But in fact, as usual, the truth is a bit more complex than it seems.

Arachidonic acid is a necessary substance for health. It is found in significant amounts in the brain and liver, and it is found in large amounts in muscles. In fact, it is often used as a nutritional supplement by body builders because of its significance in muscles.

Apart from being found in brain, liver, and muscles, arachidonic acid is also converted into many other substances in the body. Some of those substances are inflammatory, but they are essential for immune response in some cases. So a deficiency of arachidonic acid could theoretically impair immunity. At the same time, many of the substances are anti-inflammatory. On the whole, in fact, it seems that the overall effect of arachidonic acid is neutral or slightly anti-inflammatory.[12]

The suggested route by which linoleic acid might become inflammatory seems very unlikely in light of the fact that arachidonic acid isn't inflammatory. And furthermore, a review study looking at the highest quality studies investigating the subject of linoleic acid and inflammation concluded, "No evidence is available [...] that addition of [linoleic acid] to the diet increases the concentrations of inflammatory markers." [13] Unfortunately, the wording of this particular study is very specific. It doesn't state that linoleic acid doesn't increase inflammation. It just says that linoleic acid doesn't increase inflammatory *markers*. Also, the study was conducted at the University of Illinois, Urbana-Champaign at the Department of Food Science and Human Nutrition, a school that receives 46 percent of its funding from Monsanto, Syngenta, PepsiCo, Nestle, and a few other corporations you would undoubtedly recognize. So this is yet another example of a study in which it is difficult to determine whether the published results are biased by the financial interests or not. Make of it what you will.

To be honest, I haven't found much in the way of evidence that supports the claim that linoleic acid is inflammatory—at least not directly. And even though I have perpetuated that myth in other writings, I now must admit that I don't think there's good reason to think that linoleic is directly inflammatory or that even in its conversion to arachidonic acid it promotes inflammation directly.

However, there remains the fact that increases in linoleic acid in the human diet parallels the rises in cardiovascular disease, type

---

[12] Ferrucci et al. Relationship of plasma polyunsaturated fatty acids to circulating inflammatory markers. *Journal of Clinical Endocrinology and Metabolism*. 2006; 91(2): 439-446.

[13] Johnson GH and Fritsche K. Effect of dietary linoleic acid on markers of inflammation in healthy persons: a systematic review of randomized controlled trials. *Journal of the Academy of Nutrition and Dietetics*. 2012; 112(7): 1029-1041.

2 diabetes, and many other conditions that are associated with inflammation. The correlation doesn't mean that linoleic acid is the cause, but it does mean that until linoleic acid can be proven to be truly as benign (or even beneficial) as is claimed, I think it is a good idea to continue to investigate possible ways in which linoleic acid may contribute to these conditions. Furthermore, some research links high omega 6 intake with increased body fatness, [14] and increased body fatness can, in fact, increase inflammation in the body. So there may be an indirect connection.

In recent years, a great deal of interest has developed in the study of the endocannabinoid system. The prefix "endo" means internal. And "cannabi" refers to cannabis (AKA marijuana), which is the source of some of the best-studied and most famous cannabinoids such as THC—the cannabinoid known to get people "high." The exocannabinoids ("exo" meaning external) such as THC are thought to act on the endocannabinoid system. But they are not the only cannabinoids that act on the endocannabinoid system—so do natural substances produced by the human body called endocannabinoids.

Two such endocannabinoids are 2-arachidonoylglycerol (2-AG) and anandamide (also found in chocolate). Both of these are created from arachidonic acid. Although studies have found that excesses of linoleic acid don't produce excesses of arachidonic acid, it *may* be that arachidonic acid doesn't hang around but instead is converted to 2-AG and anandamide.

Dysfunction of 2-AG and anandamide signaling have been found in cases of increased body fat,[15] cardiovascular disease,[16]

[14] Muhlhausler BS and Ailhaud GP. Omega-6 polyunsaturated fatty acids and the early signs of obesity. Current opinion in endocrinology, diabetes, and obesity. 2013; 20(1): 56-61.

[15] Engeli S. Dysregulation of the endocannabinoid system in obesity. *Journal of Neuroendocrinology.* 2008; 20 Supplement 1: 110-115.

[16] Staley CP and O'Sullivan SE. Cyclooxygenase metabolism mediates vasorelaxation to 2-arachidonoylglycerol (2-AG) in human mesenteric arteries. *Pharmacological Rresearch.* 2014; 81: 74-82;.Singla et al. Cannabinoids

and possibly other conditions such as Alzheimer's disease. These endocannabinoids have been found to be important for health it isn't that 2-AG and anandamide are harmful. Not in the least. Research is now suggesting that the endocannabinoid system may be incredibly important for health. The theory is that, much as excessive dopamine release may adversely affect dopamine signaling, leading to addictions, excessive cannabinoids may adversely affect endocannabinoid signaling. The result may be health deterioration.

Interestingly, cannabinoids such as 2-AG have been found to be involved in hunger signaling. That shouldn't come as a surprise to anyone who's ever experienced "the munchies" after smoking marijuana. But when endocannabinoid signaling is thrown off, hunger signaling may be out of whack. One theory is that excessive 2-AG may cause increased eating in some cases. Simply restricting calories or exercising more won't solve the problem and will likely produce increased stress, which creates a vicious cycle of restriction and bingeing well known to the countless yo-yo dieters who have tried to achieve sustainable fat loss without success.

So although linoleic acid may not directly cause problems, it *may* indirectly lead to endocannabinoid system dysregulation. And *that* may be problematic.

Something like endocannabinoid signaling or the fate of dietary linoleic acid is incredibly complex. So, to be clear, I am merely saying that preliminary research indicates that excessive dietary linoleic acid *may* adversely alter endocannabinoid signaling, and that may cause some of the health problems. The research in this area is still very new, and the evidence in support of this theory is minimal. Much more study will be necessary to test the theory and either disprove it or support it. We'll look at a little bit more evidence shortly. But first, let's look at omega 3 fatty acids.

---

and atherosclerotic coronary heart disease. *Clinical Cardiology.* 2012; 35(6): 329-335.

Omega 3

Omega 3 fatty acids make up the other group of polyunsaturated fats. However, whereas there is a great deal of scrutiny regarding the health claims of omega 6 fatty acids, very little scrutiny is given to omega 3 fatty acids. As we'll see, omega 3 fatty acids are almost universally praised as being health promoting without any negative health consequences. Is it true? Let's take a look.

As with omega 6 fatty acids, there are lot of different types of omega 3 fatty acids, but there are only a few that are considered to be particularly important in the human diet. In fact, only one is officially considered to be essential. It is essential both in that it is considered necessary for health *and* an in that the body cannot synthesize it. That fatty acid is called alpha-linolenic acid (there's an extra 'n' in there so it's linole*n*ic acid).

Alpha-linolenic acid is found, like linoleic acid, primarily in nuts and seeds and, to a lesser extent, in the fats of the animals who eat lots of nuts and seeds. Most nuts and seeds contain large amounts of linoleic acid with very small amounts of alpha-linolenic acid. Notable exceptions are flax (58 percent) and chia (64 percent) as well as sea buckthorn (32 percent), hemp (20 percent), and walnut (10 percent).

Although alpha-linolenic acid is considered to be essential, the recommended amounts for adults are much lower than those of linoleic acid. The National Academy of Sciences suggests 1.6

grams for men and 1.1 grams for women. But like the recommendations for linoleic acid, these values are also based on average reported intakes for healthy adults rather than on rigorous studies attempting to determine how much is actually needed.

Although the amounts of alpha-linolenic acid recommended are fairly small, keep in mind that the amounts of alpha-linolenic acid found in traditional foods are much smaller than the amounts of linoleic acid, generally speaking. It's not clear that humans have traditionally eaten much flax or chia seed. And if you've ever hulled and shelled walnuts by hand using primitive tools (e.g., rocks), you probably suspect as do I that walnuts probably haven't made up a significant portion of most people's diets throughout human history.

So as with linoleic acid, chances are that most of our human ancestors had deficiencies in alpha-linoleic acid according to these standards. Could it be that the recommendations are higher than necessary?

What is the fate of alpha-linolenic acid in the body? Well, it turns out that despite being considered an essential fatty acid (in part because it cannot be synthesized and in part because it is theoretically needed), I haven't found any studies demonstrating that a deficiency is possible. Instead, all evidence is that alpha-linolenic acid is needed *primarily in the absence of dietary sources of eicosapentaenoic acid (EPA) and docosahexaenoic acid (DHA)*.[17] The body is capable of converting alpha-linolenic acid into EPA and then EPA into DHA. So if EPA and DHA are deficient in the diet, alpha-linolenic acid is necessary because EPA and DHA are necessary for health. DHA is one of the most abundant substances in the brain, for example. But the conversion rate of alpha-linolenic acid to DHA is very, very poor. It would seem that dietary sources of EPA and DHA are a much more efficient

---

[17] Gebauer et al. n-3 fatty acids dietary recommendations and food sources to achieve essentiality and cardiovascular benefits. *American Journal of Clinical Nutrition*. 2006; 83(6): S1526-S1535.

way to obtain the nutrients. Not only that, but alpha-linolenic acid has been (weakly) linked to prostate cancer, indicating that it may be *safer* to obtain EPA and DHA directly from the diet rather than through (poor) conversion from alpha-linolenic acid.

EPA and DHA are found most abundantly in fish oil, which is one of the reasons that many people believe that eating oily fish or taking fish oil supplements may be beneficial. And it certainly seems that humans have evolved eating oily fish or at least the oily parts of non-oily fish (fish heads, livers, etc.) for a very long time. So eating fish may be a reasonable suggestion. On the other hand, many humans have *not* relied extensively on fish as a food source throughout history. And so we might suspect that there's something a little... *fishy* about the suggestion that one has to either eat handfuls of flaxseeds or fish oil every day to stay healthy. It turns out that other animal foods also contain modest amounts of EPA and DHA. Eggs and meat provide EPA and DHA. Not surprisingly, many of the organ meats are high in these substances, particularly the brain, which is a traditional food that is rarely eaten in modern society (and with the current fears of so-called "mad cow disease" it's unlikely to become popular any time soon). Eating only muscle meat of grain-fed animals without also eating organs high EPA/DHA will probably lead to a deficiency. That's just a guess on my part since I haven't seen this matter studied (almost all the research is with flaxseed oil or fish oil). So there may be problems with the conventional diet of many Westerners these days and adding fish oil *may* correct that. But as we'll see shortly, I'm not convinced that it's a great idea without also making some other adjustments. And regarding flax or chia oils as alpha-linolenic acid supplements, I don't think that science supports that as an ideal solution. Again, remember that alpha-linolenic acid itself isn't clearly necessary in significant amounts. Rather, the EPA and DHA that can be the end products of alpha-linolenic acid conversion are what are needed, and the conversion rate from alpha-linolenic acid is extremely poor—estimated to be less than 1 percent conversion to DHA.

Science and popular media are currently experiencing a love affair with omega 3s, and it's easy to see why. The research into omega 3s makes them look like, if you'll pardon the somewhat inappropriate expression, the best thing since sliced bread. There are literally tens of thousands of studies into the potential benefits of omega 3s. And the results paint a very rosy picture, indeed. Looking at the studies without any context, it would be easy to believe that slamming down fistfuls of fish oil capsules can protect you from just about anything. Many studies claim to show that omega 3 supplementation or high intake of oily fish correlates with a reduction in cardiovascular disease,[18] cancer,[19] Alzheimer's,[20] Parkinson's,[21] and lots of the other big, bad, scary things that we all want to be protected from.

But the picture isn't actually quite as clear as the popular media and many book authors make it out to be. Despite the fact that increasing omega 3 intake is correlated with lots of positive outcomes, there are some negatives as well that don't typically get reported.

Omega 3 supplementation can sometimes (though not always) *reduce* insulin sensitivity and *worsen* blood sugar control.[22] Omega 3 supplementation can also increase the risk of bleeding strokes and reduce immunity due to its blood thinning capabilities.

These negatives typically only occur with relatively large amounts of supplemental fish oil in the range of 3 grams per day.

---

[18] Kris-Etherton et al. Fish consumption, fish oil, omega-3 fatty acids, and cardiovascular disease. *Circulation.* 2002; 106: 2747-2757.

[19] Jing et al. Omega-3 polyunsaturated fatty acids and cancer. *Anticancer Agents in Medicinal Chemistry.* 2013; 13(8): 1162-1177.

[20] Calon F. Omega-3 polyunsaturated fatty acids in Alzheimer's disease: key questions and partial answers. *Current Alzheimer Research.* 2011; 8(5): 470-478.

[21] Bousquet et al. Impact of omega-3 fatty acids in Parkinson's disease. *Ageing Research Reviews.* 2011; 10(4): 453-463.

[22] Glauber et al. Adverse metabolic effect of omega-3 fatty acids in non-insulin-dependent diabetes mellitus. *Annals of Internal Medicine.* 1988; 108(5): 663-668.

There is some evidence that some populations such as Alaskan natives have adapted to high omega 3 intake and have more problems with lower intake than they do with high intake. But for the rest of the population, high omega 3 intake can have negative consequences.

But even *modest* omega 3 supplementation is now linked to health problems. For example, a recent human trial showed that among men, higher omega 3 intake correlates with increased risk of prostate cancer. [23] Plus, studies are now showing that the cardiovascular protective effects of omega 3 fats may be non-existent.[24]

Although fish oil supplements remain the most popular dietary supplement in North America, some researchers are beginning to question whether more omega 3 is always the best idea. Yes, the results of omega 3 supplementation are sometimes impressive compared to controls for *some* conditions such as Alzheimer's. But because increasing omega 3 intake can have some negative consequences, some are beginning to ask whether absolute intake of omega 3 is the key or if it might be the *ratio* of omega 3 to omega 6 that matters.

---

[23] Brasky et al. Plasma Phospholipid Fatty Acids and Prostate Cancer Risk in the SELECT Trial. *Journal of the National Cancer Institute.* 2013. djt174

[24] Evangelos et al. Association Between Omega 3 Fatty Acid Supplementation and Risk of Major Cardiovascular Disease Events. *Journal of the American Medical Association.* 2012; 308(10): 1024-1033.

The Ratio

Many proponents of so-called "ancestral diets" claim that for the majority of human history we have evolved in the context of a diet that has had an omega 6 to omega 3 ratio of close to 1:1. Depending on which estimates you believe, current dietary averages for omega 6 to omega 3 ratios are between 17:1 and 30:1. Obviously, the *ratio* of omega 6 to omega 3 has changed dramatically, and many researchers are wondering if perhaps the ratio between these polyunsaturated fats might be the key to understanding the health effects.

Some prominent health researchers and personalities have outright rejected the idea that the ratio of omega 6 to omega 3 plays any role whatsoever in human health. For example, Walter Willett, the chair of the department of nutrition at the Harvard School of Public Health, has criticized the idea.[25] He claims that attempts to lower the omega 6 to omega 3 ratio will lead to increases in cardiovascular disease. He's a smart guy who is in touch with the pulse of current research, and so we would be foolish to dismiss his warnings without further investigation. But let's look a bit closer and see what we find.

It turns out that not all researchers agree with Willett's conclusions. Although there is, as we've seen, a body of evidence

---

[25] Willett WC. The role of dietary n-6 fatty acids in prevention of cardiovascular disease. *Journal of Cardiovascular Medicine*. 2007; 8 Supplement 1: S42-S45.

that suggests a "modest benefit" of high omega 6 intake, there also exists a fair amount of research showing that when the omega 6 to omega 3 ratio is elevated, there are links to worsening inflammation and higher death risk, [26] cognitive decline and Alzheimer's,[27] and cancer.[28] And other links have been made to non-alcoholic fatty liver disease, cardiovascular disease, inflammatory bowel disease, and rheumatoid arthritis.[29]

One of the ideas that is emerging from research is that changes in omega 3 status have a more significant impact on health than do similar changes in omega 6 status. And in general, relative increases in omega 3 status will have positive effects on health. The implication of this research is that instead of adding *more* omega 3s to a diet that is high in omega 6, it may be more beneficial to simply reduce the levels of omega 6. In fact, research shows that simply lowering the amount of omega 6 in the human diet (without making any changes to dietary intake of omega 3) will actually increase the levels of omega 3 in the blood.[30]

But what about Willett's warning that lowering omega 6 intake will increase cardiovascular disease risk? Well, Willett's well-informed interpretation of the evidence isn't the only valid one.

---

[26] Noori et al. Dietary omega-3 fatty acid, ratio of omega-6 to omega-3 intake, inflammation, and survival in long-term hemodialysis patients. *American Journal of Kidney Disease*. 2011; 58(2): 248-256.

[27] Leof M and Walach H. The omega-6/omega-3 ratio and dementia or cognitive decline: a systematic review on human studies and biological evidence. *Journal of Nutrition in Gerontology and Geriatrics*. 2013; 32(1): 1-23.

[28] Kang JX and Liu A. The role of the tissue omega-6/omega-3 fatty acid ratio in regulation of tumor angiogenesis. *Cancer Metastasis Reviews*. 2013; 32(1-2): 201-210.

[29] Patterson et al. Health implications of high dietary omega-6 polyunsaturated fatty acids. *Journal of Nutrition and Metabolism*. 2012; Article ID 539426, 16 pages.

[30] Wood et al. A low omega-6 polyunsaturated fatty acid (n-6 PUFA) diet increases omega-3 (n-3) long chain PUFA status in plasma phospholipids in humans. Prostaglandins, leukotrienes, and essential fatty acids. 2014; 90(4): 133-138.

For example, an Icelandic research team has found that when you replace omega 6 fats with omega 3 fats in the diet, cardiovascular risk is *lower* and survival rates in case of cardiovascular events (heart attacks, strokes, etc.) are *higher*.[31] Not a lot of human studies have looked at this matter, but some have, such as the OPTILIP study, a major British study investigating the optimal ratios of omega 6 to omega 3. The findings of that study were that reducing the omega 6 to omega 3 ratio improves cardiovascular health.[32] And one of the researchers from that study has written that the study supports the recommendation to *reduce linoleic acid intake.*[33]

There's more. Remember how endocannabinoid dysregulation and elevated levels of endocannabinoids (particularly 2-AG) are associated with a bunch of problems, including cardiovascular disease, increased fat mass, and diabetes? Well, researchers have found that it is possible to reduce the level of 2-AG in humans and potentially improve endocannabinoid signaling through dietary interventions. In particular, dramatically reducing the omega 6 to omega 3 ratio in the diet can have this effect. While reducing omega 6 intake will increase omega 3 levels in the blood, only when also adding omega 3 to the diet to further reduce the omega 6 to omega 3 ratio will arachidonic acid levels and 2-AG levels drop.[34]

---

[31] Gudbjarnason et al. Effects of n-3 polyunsaturated fatty acids on coronary heart disease. *Bibliotheca Nutritio et Dieta*. 1989; 43: 1-12.

[32] Sanders et al. Effect of varying the ratio of n-6 to n-3 fatty acids by increasing the dietary intake of alpha-linolenic acid, eicosapentaenoic and docosahexaenoic acid, or both on fibrinogen and clotting factors VII and XII in persons aged 45-70 y: the OPTILIP study. *American Journal of Clinical Nutrition*. 2006; 84(3): 513-522.

[33] Griffin BA. How relevant is the ratio of dietary n-6 to n-3 polyunsaturated fatty acids to cardiovascular disease risk? Evidence from the OPTILIP study. *Current Opinion in Lipidology*. 2008; 19(1): 57-62.

[34] Taha et al. Dietary omega-6 fatty acid lowering increases bioavailability of omega-3 polyunsaturated fatty acids in human plasma lipid pools. Prostaglandins, leukotrienes, and essential fatty acids. 2014; 90(5): 151-157.Di Marzo et al. Changes in plasma endocannabinoid levels in viscerally

In conclusion, while there is evidence of "modest benefits" to be had by increasing omega 6 (and likely the omega 6 to omega 3 ratio), there is also mounting evidence that despite Willett's warnings, lowering the omega 6 to omega 3 ratio by reducing omega 6 intake may provide greater benefits. This idea is further reinforced, but certainly not proven, by the fact that the increase in omega 6 to omega 3 ratio has paralleled the increases in cardiovascular disease and diabetes. We can't draw certain conclusions from the evidence we now have, but my hunch is that reducing omega 6 intake is the way to go.

When omega 6 intake is reduced significantly, the amount of omega 3 needed to balance omega 6 is much lower, reducing the potentially harmful effects of too much omega 3.

---

obese men following a 1 year lifestyle modification programme and waist circumference reduction: associations with changes in metabolic risk factors. *Diabetologia*. 2009; 52(2): 213-217.

Saturated Fat

As we learned earlier, the American Heart Association began to endorse the idea that saturated fat was harmful to human health starting in the early 1960s. Soon thereafter, other health advocacy organizations and governments began making similar recommendations. As of this writing, the governments and major health advocacy organizations of the U.S., Canada, Europe, the U.K., and the United Nations recommend reducing saturated fat intake and substituting polyunsaturated fats in order to reduce health risk. But are they right? Let's take a look.

The governments and organizations that recommend reducing saturated fat intake and substituting polyunsaturated fat in place of saturated fat aren't making those recommendations willy-nilly. There is considerable evidence in support of the idea that reducing saturated fat and replacing it with polyunsaturated fat can reduce cardiovascular disease risk by a small amount. And a number of systematic reviews of the available studies have shown a "small reduction in cardiovascular risk." [35] Some of those

---

[35] Hooper et al. Reduced or modified dietary fat for preventing cardiovascular disease. Cochrane System Database of Systematic Reviews. 2012; 5: CD002137.Mozaffarian et al. Effects on coronary heart disease of increasing polyunsaturated fat in place of saturated fat: a systematic review and meta-analysis of randomized controlled trials. *PLOS Medicine.* 2010; 7(3): e1000252.

Schwab et al. Effect of the amount and type of dietary fat on cardiometabolic risk factors and risk of developing type-2 diabetes,

reviews found a modest reduction in risk of death from cardiovascular disease by reducing saturated fat while others found no reduction in risk of death from cardiovascular disease.

However, for every systematic review that concludes that a small risk reduction can be had by replacing saturated fats with polyunsaturated fats, there is another that draws a different conclusion. For example, a major review from the Harvard School of Public Health concluded that the greatest risk factors for preventable death in the United States include smoking, high blood pressure, low omega 3 intake, and trans fat intake. [36] Saturated fat was not found to be a significant factor.

A systematic review published in 2014 concluded that "[c]urrent evidence does not clearly support cardiovascular guidelines that encourage high consumption of polyunsaturated fatty acids and low consumption of total saturated fats.."[37] This review drew sharp criticism from the likes of Walter Willett. In fact, Willett wrote a letter in which he claimed that the review involved multiple errors. He even went so far as to call the research "shoddy" and call for a retraction. One of Willett's own colleagues at the Harvard School of Public Health, Dr. Mozaffarian (one of the authors of the paper defending the AHA position on high omega 6 intake) was a member of the team that put together the 2014 review and Mozaffarian was far more gracious in *his* statements about the study. He said that although the conclusions of the study run contrary to his personal opinion, "science is not a dictatorship." In other words, let the data speak for itself. And in the case of this review, the data shows no

cardiovascular disease, and cancer: a systematic review. *Food and Nutrition Research*. 2014; 58.

[36] Danaei et al. The preventable causes of death in the United States: a comparative risk assessment of dietary, lifestyle, and metabolic risk factors. *PLOS Medicine*. 2009; 6(4): e1000058.

[37] Chowdhury et al. Association of dietary, circulating, and supplement fatty acids with coronary risk: a systematic review and meta-analysis. *Annals of Internal Medicine*. 2014; 160(6).

significant connection between saturated fat intake and cardiovascular disease.

Another study coming from the University of Illinois went so far as to exonerate saturated fat and instead place the blame on excess omega 6 fatty acids.[38] The author of that paper claims that excess seed oil consumption and smoking are the major contributors to cardiovascular disease by causing oxidation of cholesterol.

Individual studies demonstrate similar findings. For example, the Oslo Diet-Heart Study found that a dietary intervention that replaces saturated fat with polyunsaturated fat resulted in an increase in deaths from cardiovascular disease.[39]

Then we're left with facts that don't fit the leading theory very neatly. The leading theory says that replacing saturated fat with polyunsaturated fat (but not carbohydrates) will lower cardiovascular disease risk. However, there are troublesome examples of cultures that defy that theory. For example, the famous French paradox is that while the French people eat more saturated fat (and less seed oil) than do populations like the United States, they have *lower* rates of cardiovascular disease—some of the lowest among so-called "developed" nations.

There are also numerous examples of cultures that eat a traditional diet high in saturated fat and low in omega 6 fatty acids and have exceptionally low rates of cardiovascular disease, diabetes, and cancer. For example, some groups of Pacific islanders have found that, despite their sometimes extremely high intake of saturated fats (in some cases up to 50 percent of calories), many of the diseases blamed on saturated fat are non-existent in those populations.

---

[38] Kummerow FA. Interaction between sphingomyelin and oxysterols contributes to atherosclerosis and sudden death. *American Journal of Cardiovascular Disease*. 2013; 3(1): 17-26.

[39] Leren P. The Oslo Diet-Heart Study: eleven-year report. *Circulation*. 1970; 42: 935-942.

And then we have examples that show that dramatic reductions in saturated fat intake together with high intake of omega 6 fatty acids (matching the recommendations perfectly) do not necessarily result in lowered cardiovascular risk. As mentioned earlier, Israel has one of the highest intakes of omega 6 in place of saturated fat in the world and yet also has one of the highest rates of cardiovascular disease.

At least one study co-authored rather oddly by none other than Walter Willett (then a lowly professor) suggests that saturated fat intake is not a risk factor for cardiovascular disease. In the study, the authors found that the evidence didn't support the claim that saturated fat increased cardiovascular disease risk.[40] Rather, the authors found that high saturated fat intake was often associated with low *fiber* intake—likely meaning a lack of fresh fruits and vegetables—and that low fiber intake (or perhaps low intake of fruits and vegetables) is the more likely explanation for increased cardiovascular disease risk.

---

[40] Ascherio et al. Dietary fat and risk of coronary heart disease in men: cohort follow up study in the United States. *British Medical Journal.* 1996; 313: 84.

High Fat, Low Fat

Over the years, we've probably all heard recommendations to follow a low-fat diet at some point or another. Examples of popular low-fat diets include Pritikin, McDougall, and Ornish diets. On the other hand, we have people and organizations who recommend the opposite extreme: a low-carbohydrate, high-fat diet. Popular examples include Atkins, South Beach, and the "fat adapted" and ketogenic camps of the paleo diets.

But who's right and who's wrong? Surely, *either* low fat or high fat is superior for health while the other is clearly negative. Right? Well, let's take a look.

Some of the leading proponents of low-fat diets for health are Dean Ornish, John McDougall, and Neal Barnard. Each has written eloquently espousing the benefits of their approaches to health. And, what is more, each has been able to show that their approaches, as well as the approach of similar programs such as the Pritikin program, do seem to have potentially beneficial outcomes. And they are now famous for having inspired Bill Clinton to make dramatic dietary changes in 2010 after he had heart surgery.

While the low-fat diet gurus may make some convincing arguments, their programs are sufficiently complex that it is impossible for anyone to pinpoint precisely what about their programs may be beneficial for some people. All of them advocate for a largely plant-based, whole food diet, with some advocating for strict veganism. Also included in the programs are things such as meditation, yoga, smoking cessation, exercise, and other lifestyle changes. With all those changes, are the benefits of the programs due to the diets being low fat? How can we know?

We've already seen that Walter Willett co-authored a study that suggested that saturated fat was not problematic. Instead, the authors believed that low fiber diets were the problem, and I suspect that fiber itself isn't necessarily the missing ingredient, but rather the total nutrition obtained from foods that naturally contain substantial fiber such as fruits and vegetables. The "low-fat" diets that show benefits never advocate for replacing fat with refined starch and sugar. Instead, they advocate for whole foods such as fruits and vegetables. Therefore, necessarily, anyone following one of those "low-fat" diets will be increasing his or her intake of both fiber and nutrients from whole foods, which we already have reason to suspect will lower cardiovascular disease risk (and risk of just about every disease) in and of itself, completely independent of dietary fat in the diet.

Smoking, poor stress management, and lack of exercise are all well established as *major* risk factors for a long list of diseases. So any program that effectively causes participants to stop smoking, manage stress more effectively, and move more will reduce their risk of nearly all diseases. And that benefit is completely independent of dietary fat.

So despite the fact that many of the low-fat diet gurus can demonstrate health improvements among those who can successfully follow the programs (which also demonstrates a sincere commitment on the part of the individual to improve his or her health, which also contributes to success in improving health), there still is no evidence that lowering total fat intake will lower risk of disease.

On the other hand, we have ample evidence from those who follow extreme low-carbohydrate, high-fat diets that those diets can *also* promote health improvements *when in the context of overall lifestyle changes*. This is evidenced by the popularity of low carbohydrate, high fat websites on which people share their success stories in which they lean out, gain energy, improve fasting glucose levels, reverse cardiovascular disease, and so forth. They often attribute the positive changes to eating a low-carbohydrate, high-fat diet. But, of course, like those who follow the low-fat dietary programs, those on the high-fat programs generally are also making so many changes in their lives that it is impossible to pinpoint the exact cause or causes of any health benefits.

Fortunately, research can shed some light on this subject. The research shows that *both* low-fat *and* high-fat diets can work equally well for *short-term* weight loss.[41] Ketogenic diets (very low carbohydrate, low protein, very high fat) have been shown to have therapeutic value in some conditions such as epilepsy.[42] But when it comes to disease risk, neither seems to make much difference.[43]

There are some troubles with both extremes, however. Diets very high in fat are— pardon me for saying so—disgusting. I'm not talking about eating lots of butter on mashed potatoes, for example. That's delicious. But rather, I'm talking about diets in which carbohydrate intake is extremely low and fats are extremely

[41] Nordmann et al. Effects of low-carbohydrate versus low-fat diets on weight loss and cardiovascular risk factors. *Archives of Internal Medicine*. 2006; 166(3): 285-293. Meckling et al. Comparison of a low fat diet to a low carbohydrate diet on weight loss, body composition, and risk factors for diabetes and cardiovascular disease in free-living, overweight men and women. *Journal of Clinical Endocrinology and Metabolism*. 2013; 89(6).

[42] Paoli et al. Beyond weight loss: a review of therapeutic uses of very-low-carbohydrate (ketogenic) diets. *European Journal of Clinical Nutrition*. 2013; 67: 789-796; Sharman et al. A ketogenic diet favorably affects serum biomarkers for cardiovascular disease in normal-weight men. *Journal of Nutrition*. 2002; 132(7): 1879-1885.

[43] Howard et al. Low fat dietary pattern and risk for cardiovascular disease: the women's health initiative randomized controlled dietary modification trial. *Journal of the American Medical Association*. 2006; 295(6): 655-666;. Burr et al. Effects of changes in fat, fish, and fibre intakes on death and myocardial reinfarction: diet and reinfarction trial (DART). *The Lancet*. 1989; 334; 757-761.

high. I like broccoli, and I like butter a lot. But I don't want broccoli *swimming* in butter. Diets very high in fat have been shown to be almost always *low-calorie* diets because no one wants to eat that much fat without carbohydrates.

Low-calorie diets aren't sustainable in the long run. If the calories in are *less* than calories out, the inevitable result is fatigue sooner or later. And if fat intake is very high and carbohydrates are low, there will be a carbohydrate deficiency with all the symptoms of that, including insomnia, irritability, anxiety, and so forth. The low-carbohydrate, "fat-adapted" party only lasts so long for most people, and when it's over, the deficiency symptoms set in, and it ain't much fun.

But as long as you eat a very high fat diet with adequate quantity and variety of low-carbohydrate vegetables, dairy, and meats, you'll probably have adequate nutrition except for the missing calories and carbohydrates. Very low-fat diets, on the other hand, depending on the extreme to which they are taken, can produce a deficiency in fat-soluble nutrients such as preformed vitamin A, vitamin K2, and vitamin E. Low-fat diets have also been shown to reduce testosterone levels and increase estrogen levels in men.[44]

So either extreme is both unnecessary and potentially harmful for most people. Unless you have epilepsy that is treatable by a ketogenic diet, chances are, a diet that includes *moderate* (not ridiculous) amounts of dietary fat along with plenty of carbohydrates is probably sensible. Studies have shown that a diet that is roughly 30 percent fat by calories is often ideal for hormone production. That's usually quite easy to eat without trying because it's normally about what tastes good.

---

[44] Dorgan et al. Effects of dietary fat and fiber on plasma and urine androgens and estrogens in men: a controlled feeding study. *American Journal of Clinical Nutrition.* 1996; 64(6): 850-855; .Hämäläinen et al. Decrease of serum total and free testosterone during a low fat high fibre diet. *Journal of Steroid Biochemistry.* 1983; 18(3): 369-370.

What the Heck Should You Eat?

We've covered a lot of information in this short book. As you can hopefully see, there are no perfectly clear and simple answers. Some studies show that omega 6 fats may be good for heart health, but then again, other studies show exactly the opposite. Likewise, some studies show a "modest benefit" from reducing saturated fat intake, but then again, plenty of other studies conclude that there is no association between saturated fat and cardiovascular disease. Smart men like Walter Willett say to follow the conventional recommendations while some of the researchers whose work has been used to justify those recommendations say that the AHA and others have misunderstood the research. What do you do? Should you gorge yourself on Kerrygold and medium chain triglyceride oil like you're livin' la vida low carb? Or should you avoid all dietary fat like the plague as Ornish and McDougall would have you do?

A lot of authors on the subject will tell you what to think and what to do. I've done that as well in some of my writing. But with this book, I want to give you the information so that you can form your own educated conclusions. I don't want to tell you what to do. And for a couple of good reasons.

For one thing, there's a very good reason why some very smart, very well-meaning people can have dramatically opposed views when it comes to nutritional matters. That's because the evidence is often conflicting. So if I tell you what the "right" thing to eat is, I'd have to be delusional. I don't know for sure any more than anyone else does. The more I learn, the more I am convinced of that.

The second reason I don't want to tell you what to eat is because if I do, I am helping to undermine your trust in the one authority that you *should* trust: your body. With so much dietary and lifestyle advice these days, it's so easy to forget that our bodies are miraculously attuned to their needs. That's not just some New Age sound bite. That's actually straight out of biology 101. In fact, one of the most respected physiologists in modern history, a guy named Walter Cannon, the chairman of the Department of Physiology at Harvard Medical School in the early 1900s—no slouch, in other words-—did much to further the notion of homeostasis, which is widely accepted among physiologists today. And Cannon so thoroughly believed in the wisdom of the body (in fact, he wrote a book titled *The Wisdom of the Body*) that he stated unequivocally that the body is always striving to maintain balance, and every impulse is in that singular interest. In other words, if you are thirsty, then you need fluids, and if you are not thirsty, you do *not* need fluids. Or, to put it into the context of this book, if you desire soy oil, then your body probably needs soy oil, but if you don't desire soy oil, you probably don't need it. (I'm willing to wager, by the way, that few humans actually crave soy oil on a regular basis. But butter on mashed potatoes? That's another story.)

So my actual hope with this book is to remove much of the "shoulds" from dietary fats so that you can simply trust your body's wisdom. Depending on where we get our dietary guidance, we've alternatively been told that we should eat or avoid saturated fat, omega 6 fat, omega 3 fat, and fat in general. As a result, we've often got a cacophony of little dietary dictators shouting at us in our heads, so to speak. But all that noise can drown out the natural promptings of the body unless we learn to tune into that wisdom.

Finally, the third reason I don't want to tell you what to eat is because that just creates more negative stress for you. And interestingly, research shows that elevated stress hormones may be *the* determining factor in whether or not you experience health *regardless* of what you eat.

Cannon, our Harvard man, actually is the one credited with coining the term "stress" as we use it to refer to our experiences in the body. And following on Cannon's work was Hans Selye, one of the 20th century's most awarded and celebrated medical professionals. Selye actually demonstrated that prolonged stress in the body—regardless of the cause, be it nutritional, emotional, environmental, physiological, or otherwise—produces the same harmful effects. And those effects look a whole lot like cardiovascular disease, diabetes, cancer, and many of the other conditions that are more commonly blamed on diet and exercise.

To be sure, diet does influence health, but it would seem that chronic stress is what makes or breaks the deal. For example, let's say that Willett is right —that eating saturated fat really will clog your arteries and give you a heart attack while seed oils will protect. (I'll admit that given the evidence we've explored in this book, I'm skeptical of this claim.) How can we explain that many people stand in stark contrast to that? Is it purely genetic? The work of Selye and many stress researchers since him suggest a different story. They suggest that when a person has a healthy stress response and maintains healthy levels of stress hormones most of the time, that person is unlikely to have a heart attack whether he eats sticks of butter or guzzles soy oil. But on the other hand, the classic Type A personality who is upset with life for being so inconvenient is just waiting for a heart attack, and he's going to need a lot more than dietary intervention to help him out.

So stressing about food turns out to be counterproductive. This is a point I've been trying to make in a roundabout manner throughout many of my books, but only now has it become so clear to me. My sincere hope is that this book has helped to remove some of the "shoulds" from your life and has done away with some of the stress about food.

With all that said, I know some of you may be dissatisfied with that conclusion. So let me share with you what *I* would do given the research presented in this book.

For my part, I simply don't see a strong argument to be made for the supposed benefits of omega 6 fats like linoleic acid in large amounts. The statistics for heart disease, for example, show that its rates have increased in parallel with increases in omega 6 fat intake, and prior to 1900, rates were pretty darn low. That was back when people were eating substantial amounts of butter, lard, and tallow—all foods that, according to the omega 6 advocates, should have been causing one massive heart attack the whole worldwide. So I'm very dubious of the health claims regarding omega 6 fats.

Taking this back home to the wisdom of the body, the simple fact is, I have absolutely no cravings for soy, corn, safflower, or canola oil. So I don't have to rely on the Harvard School of Public Health or the American Heart Association or Mark Sisson or Jimmy Moore to tell me what to do. I can just listen to my body. And if I was to put words to what my body has to say about industrial seed oils, it would be something like, "Ewwwww."

What about fish oil? Well, I happen to like salmon. Not so much that I eat it all the time. But every once in a while, I like it. I like it best with some butter, incidentally. But I don't have a hankering for liquid fish oil. So I'm doubtful that I really need to be eating it—including in encapsulated form.

When it comes to saturated fat, I also don't see any convincing arguments that it is such a bad thing. And fats like butter that have a lot of saturated fat turn out to be pretty darn delicious. I mean, I'm a potato guy. I *really* like potatoes. If I were going to play one of those silly hypothetical scenario games like being stranded on a desert island with only one food, I'd probably choose potato. That's how much I like potato. But potatoes are *way* better with some salt and ample butter. So I'm a believer in the taste (and nutritional) benefits of butter and other natural, traditional fats that happen to be fairly high in saturated fat.

Finally, high fat or low fat? I go through phases of slightly higher (maybe 60 percent of calories) and slightly lower (maybe 20 percent of calories), but tend to hover around the middle ground. Call me crazy, but I think my body knows what it needs. After all, my body is maintaining homeostasis with something like a gajillion variables at play. I can consciously remember about seven things all at once (just enough to dial a phone number). I'm going to trust my body on this one.

Of course, things change over time. And everyone is different. So I'm certainly *not* suggesting that what my body wants/needs right now is what your body needs for all time. That would be ridiculous. But I bet if you listen to your body, you'll do all right. Just ask yourself, for example, what sounds better: a baked potato with soy oil drizzled over it or a baked potato with a few pats of butter. Or how about this one: potatoes fried in corn and/or safflower oil or potatoes fried in coconut oil like potato chips used to be when I was a kid? Okay, yeah, I'm overdoing the potato thing. But you get the point.

Finally, in conclusion, as I've already suggested, diet is just one small part of the equation. Other factors that play significant roles in health include stress, movement, sunlight, relationships, hobbies and interests, smoking, and sleep. Ironically, fixation on dietary rules can backfire because it can increase stress, harm relationships, detract from hobbies and interests, and interfere with sleep quality. Most extreme dietary practices—whether very high fat, very low fat, high omega 6, high omega 3, etc.—are incompatible with full health because they tend to create food obsession.

But what if we just listen to our bodies? If you listen to your body, you can't predict what you're going to need in an hour, much less for all eternity. Talk about living in the now! Should you eat those fatty BBQ ribs? What about that salmon? Buttered corn on the cob? Or should you opt for the low-fat fruit salad instead? Your body will know in that moment.

Nutritional fads come and go, and in their wake they leave a great deal of harm. Today's conventional wisdom is held up for scorn tomorrow. And since a little bit of research scratching beneath the surface reveals that much of the evidence in support of present nutritional fads, including the dietary fat fads of all stripes, is weak, I say, trust your body's wisdom. Don't fear the food.

May you enjoy good food, good friends, and good health.

Get My Future Books FREE

If you enjoyed this book (hey, if you made it this far it couldn't have been that bad), you'll probably enjoy many of my other books about health and wellness. And you can get all my new releases in health and wellness for free by signing up for my mailing list at www.JoeyLottHealth.com. It's simple, it's free, and it's totally honest and legitimate. Nothing scammy or spammy or anything else like that (i.e., I won't be trying to sell you The 7 Dirty Underground Top Secret Weird Tricks for Rock Hard Abs or Young Living Oils). It's just about free books for those who appreciate my work, because I appreciate YOU. Simple as that.

Connect with Me

I welcome your questions, comments, and feedback of any kind. Please feel free to email me at JoeyLott@gmail.com. I am now receiving so many emails that I cannot always reply to each one, but I do read them all, and I do my best to reply to as many as possible. For the benefit of others, I may choose to publish my response to your email on my blog or in book format. I will maintain your privacy and anonymity should I choose to publish my response.

One Small Favor

My sincere goal in writing is to share something that may be of value to you. And I endeavor to do so while keeping the cost low for readers. The success of my books and my ability to reach other readers who may benefit from my books depends in large part on having lots of thoughtful, honest reviews written about my work. You would do me a great favor if you would please take a moment to generously write a review of this book on Amazon.com. This will only take a few minutes of your time, and you will be helping me a great deal. I sure would appreciate it.

About the Author

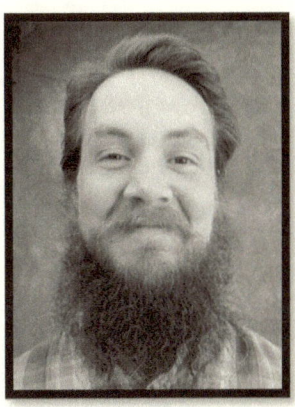

"The secret to happiness is to let go of everything—see through every assumption."

From a very young age, Joey Lott experienced intensifying anxiety. For several decades he lived with restrictive eating disorders, obsessions, compulsions, and an inescapable fear. By the time he was 30 years old, he was physically sick, emotionally volatile, and mentally obsessed with keeping any and all unwanted thoughts and experiences at bay.

At this time, Lott was living on a futon mattress in a tiny cabin in the woods. He was so sick that he could barely move. He was deeply depressed and hopeless. All of this, despite doing all the "right" things, such as years of meditation, yoga, various "perfect" diets, clean air, and pure water.

Just when things were at their most dire, a crack appeared in the conceptual world that had formerly been mistaken for reality. By peering into this crack to see underneath all of the assumptions that had been unquestioned up to that moment, Lott began a great undoing. The revelation of this undoing is that reality is utterly simple, ever present, seamless, and indivisible.

Lott's books provide a glimpse into the seamless, simple, and joyous nature of reality, offering a glimpse through the crack in conceptual worlds. Whether writing about the ultimate non-dual nature of reality, eating disorders, stress, disease, or any other subject, he offers the invitation to look at things differently. He challenges us to leave behind the old, outgrown, painful limitations we have used to bind ourselves in suffering, and then, he welcomes you home to the effortless simplicity of yourself as you are.

You can find more of Joey's books here: http://amzn.to/1bHHRRP

www.ingramcontent.com/pod-product-compliance
Lightning Source LLC
Chambersburg PA
CBHW032032290526
45786CB00012B/2593